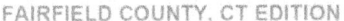

FROM
OKAY TO
FABULOUS

I0447201

10 Quick Tips to Get **Slim,
Sexy** AND Still Enjoy Your
Favorite **Comfort Foods**
And **Social Life**.

LISA CUMMINGS
The Slim and Sexy Mom's Expert

Printed in the United States of America

Warning-Disclaimer

This document is written as a source of information only. The
information contained in this document should by no means be
considered a substitute for the advice of a qualified medical
professional, who should always be consulted before beginning any new
diet or other health program. The author disclaims any liability for any
adverse effects arising from the use or application of the information
contained herein.

ABOUT LISA AND THIS BOOK

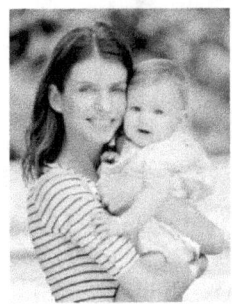

I was the type who was never overweight, but I was obsessed with the wrong foods and always on a diet. I had more of an athletic build. But just because I didn't need to lose weight from an outside perspective didn't mean I wasn't suffering on the inside. I was puffy and bloated from years of yo-yo dieting, and I over-exercised to justify overeating refined sugars and starches. I felt horrible in my clothes and I hated how I looked from age 13 to 33.

Here's the strange part – I considered myself knowledgeable about food and health all those years. But, why, then, was I overeating junk foods every chance I could? That was my madness. I would starve, overeat, then over-exercise. I didn't realize the stress I was putting on myself, not just physically, but emotionally.

Moving into a high-octane professional life in advertising didn't help things either. While my outside image seemed stable and glamorous, my inner picture of health really began to deteriorate.

I knew I needed help, but medical intervention wasn't helping. So I turned to natural healing through the power of food. And guess what? It worked.

I said farewell to my advertising career of 12 years, trained at the Institute for Integrative Nutrition (accredited by SUNY Purchase College and Cornell University), and became a member of the American Association of Drugless Practitioners (AADP). I got my Raw Foods Certification to enhance my health even further and now I share that knowledge with clients.

I have been at the same weight for over ten years now. When I wake up, I feel younger than I am, rested, physically light, free of aches and pains and best of all, I don't have to think about what drastic diet I have to go on to feel this way. This is still so amazing to me, ten years later. I owe this transition to figuring out what whole foods work best in my body for optimum health and wellness.

I love showing busy moms and their families how to integrate healthier, more cleansing foods that satisfy their daily dietary needs and hectic schedules. **Positive food choices are the key to living a sexy, happy life in a body you love.**

In this book, I share my favorite secrets and local finds that support a sound, sustainable way of eating. Eating that includes style, lots of flavor, fun and convenience. You can finally say goodbye to creeping weight gain, yo-yo dieting and pre-mature aging by applying the principles in this book to fit your unique lifestyle. Get ready to embark upon a new way of life where you can have your cake and it eat, too!

Living in Westport, Connecticut, as a health and nutrition coach has only enhanced my love of living a cleansing, sexy lifestyle even more. From the beach to the woods, to being a new mom and living in my dream home – It's just beautiful here. Being able to share what this community offers with my daughter, husband and clients brings me the kind of daily joy I never dreamed possible.

This book is dedicated to all the fabulous women in Fairfield County, Connecticut, who want to look and feel sexy – no matter what their age. I'm talking to all the busy moms, career women, empty nesters and anyone else who is tired of just getting by, feeling okay and who may not like:

- Looking in full-length mirrors

- Eating piles of dark leafy greens

- Hiding behind baggy clothes

- Juicing all day long

- Yo-yo dieting

- Obsessive calorie counting

- Giving up their favorite comfort foods

- Feeling hungry throughout the day

- Spending endless hours in the kitchen or the gym

There is a much more satisfying, and sexier way to feel lighter, leaner and look younger!

Consider this book your new BFF if you are someone who wants to:

- Get lean and sexy and stay that way

- Cleanse your body from years of toxic eating

- Enjoy cooking more, eating out and keeping your favorite comfort foods

- Make social plans without sabotaging your health goals

- Look great in a bathing suit all year long

HOW TO MAKE THIS BOOK WORK FOR YOU

This book is a **fast-track guide** for Fairfield County women, like you, to help take the fear out of doing what it takes to live a sexy lifestyle 24/7. You may ask, "How can I live a slim and sexy lifestyle without extreme dieting? Or feeling deprived? Doesn't that mean I have to juice all day, give up sweets, have a personal chef and personal trainer, and never eat out again?"

The short answer: No. But let's get clear for a second. You can do a 3-day, 5-day or 10-day all-juice cleanse, if you like, and see quick results. But please know this extreme approach will not miraculously cleanse years of overeating and accumulated waste that has built up over the years in your body's cells. This long-term waste is the culprit for unwanted belly fat, a dull complexion and lingering pounds.

The word "cleansing" is overused in our culture and often triggers negative emotions. It implies "going hungry or going without." This book offers the opposite! It's about eating clean foods, having fun, socializing, traveling and getting back in touch with real food, your true hunger patterns and learning how to satisfy them properly.

If you integrate more plant-based foods that add hydration, nutrients, and pass through the intestines efficiently, your overall health can be restored. You will **experience permanent weight loss, a boosted metabolism, glowing skin, reduction of cellulite, and a clearer, calmer mind — all with taste, style and fun!**

Yes, it's true, ladies. I will show you how to eat more organic, seasonal, whole foods for better nutrient absorption, long-term vibrancy, and balance in your body.

It's not about becoming a vegetarian, vegan or a raw foodist. Those are merely labels. This is about vegetable-centric meals combined with meat, chicken, fish, eggs, raw cheeses, grains, nuts, seeds and healthy fats for ultimate meal satisfaction.

Get ready to experience some delicious flavors, restaurants and healthy markets that are conveniently in your neighborhood. And gear up for a longer, healthier, disease-free life.

Now *that's* sexy.

WHAT YOU GET IN THIS BOOK:

1. A **Slim and Sexy Cleansing Tip** to apply to your unique lifestyle TODAY.

2. A suggested **Slim and Sexy Action Step** to make this lifestyle easily work NOW so you can experience what it feels like to live in a vibrant body, be at your ideal weight, and get fueled with a new type of energy that doesn't come from caffeine, sugar or refined flour.

3. A local **"Okay to Fabulous" Resource** to conveniently get what you need FAST whether it's at a local Whole Foods, a nearby natural cafe or market, or online. You don't have to run around all day shopping for food and spend endless hours in the kitchen or give in to junk. Make this lifestyle an easy priority with my top-picked resources that are right at your fingertips here in Fairfield County.

MOTIVATE & INSPIRE OTHERS!
"SHARE THIS BOOK"

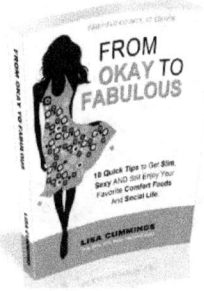

From Okay to Fabulous

10 Quick Tips to Get Slim, Sexy and Still Enjoy Your Favorite Comfort Foods and Social Life

---

Everyone deserves to look and feel sexy at any age. Lisa offers simple suggestions and local resources that will inspire you to make healthy choices and still eat what you love. Eating that involves taste, style, convenience and FUN for long-lasting results.

$9.95

To place an order, go to: **livewellbydesign.net/products**

From Okay to Fabulous

TABLE OF CONTENTS

SECTION ONE

GET SLIM AND SEXY AT ANY AGE

My clients often come to me with this belief: "I've tried many diets before that didn't work, so why should this way of eating be any different?"

Here's the good news: It's not a diet! It's a lifestyle where you get healthy and still eat what you love. You learn to eat based on a new group of foods that fit your unique tastes and bring you pleasure and results.

SLIM AND SEXY TIP #1

Focus on Progress, Not Perfection

Don't worry about getting too perfect or obsessive with your plan of eating. This is meant to be enjoyable and life enhancing, not torture.

Start by eating less processed foods. In other words, start eating more foods found in nature. It's very simple. This means you can identify where the food came from. For instance, an apple or brown rice is considered a real, whole food. One came from a tree (apple) and the other from the earth (whole grain rice). Fritos, Snickers or most baked goods, pastries and packaged foods don't come from nature. They are highly processed and create toxicity in the body.

Avoid ultimatums. After working personally with clients, I am convinced that ultimatums are a dead end road. I hear many women declare, "I'm quitting everything to lose unwanted pounds." Eventually they go back to their old eating patterns because that mentality is not sustainable.

As soon as we put a big "Forbidden Foods" list in front of our faces, we end up with bingeing, guilt trips and food obsessions. This lifestyle is about enhancing and expanding our repertoire of whole foods GRADUALLY to make better choices for pure health and enjoyment based on flavors you already love.

Action Step:
Make This Work In Your Life NOW!

When making a meal at home or when eating out at a restaurant (that preferably serves quality, fresh organic food), change just ONE thing about your order. That's progress!

Order a sweet potato with a house salad instead of having the refined pasta or french fries with unhealthy saturated fats. If white potatoes are the only thing on the menu (at many diners, for instance) order a side of roasted potatoes or a baked white potato. You don't have to eliminate your comfort foods completely, just add-in a more nutrient-dense one. Add organic butter and sea salt if you like. You'll get the same comforting feeling, minus the artificial ingredients.

When it comes time for dessert, order a soothing cup of herbal tea (bring stevia, a natural plant sweetener, in your purse for desired sweetness). Enjoy the conversations and company and look forward to a piece of dark chocolate at home. By pausing and waiting, you may even find you aren't hungry for anything else once you're home — which is one of the amazing discoveries of this lifestyle. We don't need as much food as we think.

"Okay to Fabulous" Local Resource:

Artisan
275 Old Post Rd., Southport - 203.307.4222

This chic hotspot is a delightful experience in every way. The "farm to table" New England cuisine supports sustainable, organic agriculture with its seasonally inspired dishes. Get ready to be taken away and have your taste buds come alive! There's no need to stay home and "get healthy" when you can enjoy dining out like this.

Request the outdoor patio in the summer and you'll think you're on a movie set.

I started with the fresh mesclun mix salad that came with a beet juice cocktail in a beautiful shot glass. Talk about sexy, delicious food!

The local striped bass with herbal lemon sauce, the scallops in citrus brown butter, and the grilled calamari with sweet and sour eggplant rocked my world.

And don't ignore their sides either. The Hen of the Woods mushrooms and sautéed French beans add flavor to any meal. You won't care if you didn't get your junk food fix because you will be so pleasantly full with all the harmonic robust flavors of natural, whole foods.

Eleanor Roosevelt

was so wise!

Her advice?

"You must do the

thing you think

you cannot do."

SLIM AND SEXY TIP #2

Add-In More Foods,
Don't Take Them Out

The first step to cleaning up your diet is to replace the fattening, mood-crashing, processed "junk" that has added on pounds over the years. Then add-in healthier, tastier options without turning your life upside down. The result? A stimulated metabolism, increased focus and energy, and less mood swings.

Action Step:
Make This Work In Your Life NOW!

Instead of removing all of your favorite junk foods at once, try adding in more of the right kinds of foods first. Then you'll see that your cravings for processed foods will decrease. Sounds strange, right? Add in more foods to crave less? This is one of the many joys of clean eating. It's not about less, it's about more nutritious, flavorful foods.

For instance, it's amazing what happens when vegetables like cauliflower (my favorite) roast in their own juices for 25 minutes. With some olive oil and sea salt in a 350-degree oven, they taste heavenly. I'm not joking — they taste like crispy french fries! Add vegetables like this on top of a giant salad or as a side to a piece of fish, and you will see how dinners come alive and satisfy you more.

Try dipping the crispy roasted cauliflower in organic ketchup and you've created a healthy "diner style" meal at home.

Roasting works with many other vegetables (cut them in small pieces, chunks or strips, then bake with sea salt and olive oil):

- butternut squash
- Brussels sprouts
- broccoli
- eggplant
- sweet potatoes
- parsnips (cut them in circles about 1/4 inch thick, bake until they are crunchy, and you'll have healthy croutons!)

You'll fall in love with vegetables all over again and wonder why you ever left them behind in the first place.

"Okay to Fabulous" Local Resource:

The Dressing Room
27 Powers Court, Westport - 203.226.1114

This is another one of my favorite local, homegrown, organic spots where I bring family, meet other moms (with our babies) for lunch or go there for "date night" with my husband. I recommend their caramelized Brussels sprouts as a delicious side to another appetizer or main dish. It's the perfect balance of salt, crunch and tenderness.

The key to vibrant health is to NOT fill up on heavy refined breads before dinner or dense desserts with refined sugar after dinner (unless of course it's a special occasion and you really feel like it). Remember that overindulging on foods that aren't nutrient-dense or hydrating has its consequences. It slows down digestion, contains very little enzymes, water or nutrients, and adds on weight over time.

Instead, fill up on a health-generating organic green salad with a tangy vinaigrette before your meal. Add volume to your dinner with the roasted Brussels sprouts as a side or whole grain rice if available. Feel free to order another serving of veggies if you're really hungry! You won't regret that choice in the morning when you're bouncing out of bed with lots of clear-headed energy and a flat tummy.

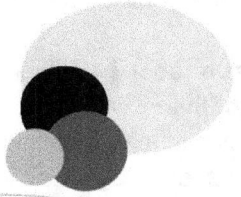

"When I started this lifestyle, I was a bit skeptical. But then my energy levels increased, I lost weight and my skin improved dramatically; I feel and look younger! Bringing clean foods into my lifestyle has given me and my family a new outlook on food and life."

~ *Kelly F., Client, Mom, Financial Analyst, Boston, MA*

SLIM AND SEXY TIP #3

Master Healthy Eating On-the-Go

What happens to your clean eating when you're on-the-go, living your life? For most people, this is where they hit the pitfalls and fall back into old eating patterns that sabotage their success. Instead, navigate specific challenges unique to your lifestyle by PLANNING AHEAD when you're:

- traveling
- celebrating birthdays
- enjoying the holidays
- dining out
- dealing with food sensitivities
- eating at work

Remember, failing to plan is planning to fail.

Action Step:
Make This Work In Your Life NOW!

Try this trick when eating out: Use the "plan, scan, or can" technique. Beforehand, decide on a food **PLAN**—for example, that you'll start with a fiber-rich salad or vegetable-based soup. Looking at the menu ahead of time online helps you easily plan and prepare so there are no big surprises or temptations.

When the waiter hands you the menu, give it a cursory **SCAN** to hone in on your choices, and ignore everything else. (Once you lock in on the fettuccine Alfredo, it can be tough to resist.)

If you want to order a favorite, less nutritious dish, make your selection healthier by asking, '**CAN** I have steamed veggies instead of fries?' or 'Can you grill the fish tacos rather than fry them?'" You will be amazed how your servers are willing to accommodate you if you politely ask for some minor adjustments based on what is already on the menu.

Try this trick when you're invited to someone's house for dinner: Offer to bring a dish. Make it exactly the way you like it, so at least you know there is something there that suits your tastes. Chances are people will love it and ask what's in it. If they don't, we don't take anything personally in this lifestyle. We eat this way because we love how it makes us look and feel.

"Okay to Fabulous" Local Resource:

Happy Cow
A Healthy Eating Food Finder - www.happycow.net

I use this incredibly handy online resource to make sure I am living a cleansing, sexy lifestyle no matter where I am. Whether I'm going home for a visit, just a few hours away, across the country, or traveling internationally, there's nothing worse than feeling bloated, blocked, and out of sorts when eating foods that don't agree with you.

You'll be amazed how many healthy spots exist to support this way of life. I found a delicious organic restaurant in Worcester, Massachusetts that's nestled amongst pizza places and bagel shops. Who knew?

Simply go to the site and key in the zip code for your destination or hotel, and there you have it. You'll get a list of local addresses of health food stores, juice bars and vegetarian choices at your fingertips that serve healthy, vibrant foods to stay nourished and energized wherever you are.

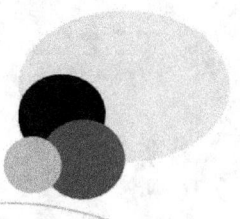

"This lifestyle is very easy, even when I commute into New York City three days a week. I've lost four pounds already and my 3PM cookie craving has disappeared just by adding in better quality foods as part of my main meals."

~ *Mary K., Client, Mom, Human Resources Director, New York City*

SECTION TWO

FIND
YOUR OWN
LEVEL OF
FABULOUSNESS

Many women say to me: "Getting healthy and living this fabulous life is going to take so much work and time!" And I say, "Doesn't it take a lot of work and time to go on fad diets, determine how much you will undereat or overeat, and obsess about your weight year after year?

If you stick to foods you recognize in nature and season them to your liking with ease and confidence, you will soon begin to crave more real foods and flavors without lots of heavy sauces and artificial boosts. You may even crave a yoga class, or even a brisk walk outside. How fabulous would that be?

SLIM AND SEXY TIP #4

Gain Confidence in the Kitchen
Even If You Don't Know How To Cook

Whether you're a foodie and love to cook, or you prefer assembling quick meals (like me), or even if you're brand new to what happens in a kitchen, take control of your health and the wellness of your loved ones by setting up your kitchen with flavor enhancing condiments and products that inspire clean choices day in and day out.

Action Step:
Make This Work In Your Life NOW!

Fill your cupboards with things like olive oil, sea salt, avocados, soy sauce, raw nuts, pure maple syrup, organic butter, dried fruits, vinegars, tahini, herbs, spices... and yes, even wine and dark chocolate!

These foods help make weeknight meals easy and satisfying. Wake up energized and lean when you add real flavors to your meals to meet your demanding palette. When you start with pure food, you don't need to add much to make it taste great.

> **Try this for a quick, creamy dip that can also be used as a salad dressing:** Take a red pepper, a few tablespoons olive oil, one avocado, sea salt, the juice of one lemon and a dash of cayenne pepper and cumin. Cut veggies and avocado into chunks and blend all ingredients in a high-speed blender. Enjoy!

Double L Market and "Lloyd"
730 Post Rd., Westport - 203.557.4705

When I moved from NYC to Westport, I was worried I wouldn't find quality, local, organic food — and then I discovered the Double L! It's like an outdoor farm stand, only indoors with beautiful produce that you'll want to pick up, smell, touch and sample each week.

You'll get to know Lloyd, who greets you with a smile every visit. He loves talking about the first seasonal deliveries of the day, like nectarines from Amish Country, peaches or strawberries. Just being there, you'll get to know more about the farmers in our area and a few cooking suggestions from Lloyd himself.

My daughter loves going with me. Lloyd carries her around and feeds her blackberries and raspberries.

A few of my favorites are his salmon from Canada. The best I've ever tasted! His salad greens, kirby cucumbers, heirloom tomatoes, sweet corn, honeydew melons and cotton candy grapes are a must-have in our kitchen. He also carries products from local vendors, like homemade salad dressings, maple syrups, quiches and artisanal cheeses.

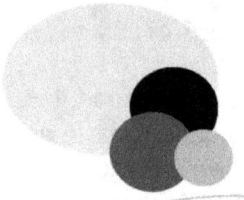

"Guess what! I made the adzuki beans with coconut and loved them. I'm making the meatloaf tonight from the cookbook you gave me. I even bought organic bison meat to try. Spent some time checking out new foods in the health food store now that I know how to read labels – can't wait to experiment with them this week".

~ *Amy M., Client, Financial Software Sales, New York City*

SLIM AND SEXY TIP #5

Feed Your Soul Cravings

One of the biggest secrets to fast-tracking your health results is upgrading what nourishes you beyond what comes on your plate. Not only will your physical body improve, your career, relationships, exercise, and life-balance improves, too, when you understand the connection between what you put in your mouth and what truly nourishes your soul.

Action Step:
Make This Work In Your Life NOW!

Nutrition comes from many factors in addition to food. Spend time outdoors in the sunlight, enjoy the company of family and friends, take outdoor hikes, meditate, build supportive relationships, work in a satisfying career, take classes that interest you, and exercise in ways that are fun. All of these things contribute to less stress, a sense of freedom, ease, and connection with your life and your body. This means less emotional eating or eating out of boredom.

Discover what you love beyond your plate.

Here are a few ideas to get you started:

- Sign up for a Zumba, dance, spinning or yoga class in your area
- Plan a weekend away and really allow yourself to unplug

- Clean out a drawer or closet
- Spend time with a friend you haven't seen in a while
- Book a massage, manicure or pedicure (and get the extra-long foot massage!)
- Take a walk on the beach

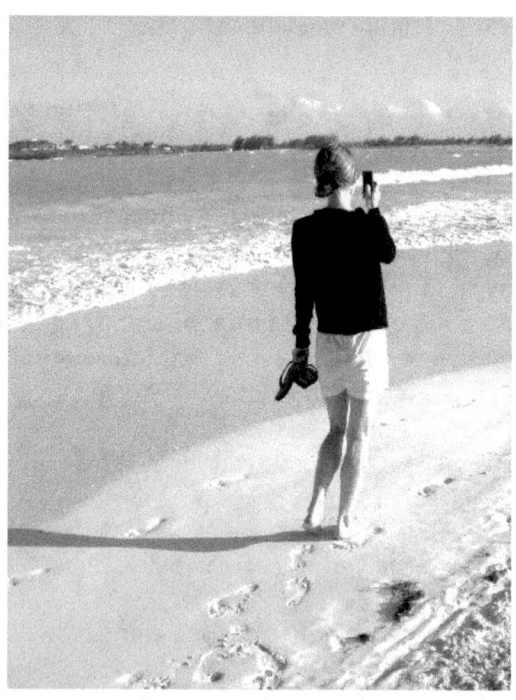

"Okay to Fabulous" Local Resource:

Intensity Fitness and Tennis

490 Westport Ave., Norwalk - 203.853.7727

I joined this privately owned fitness center when I was looking for a place to unwind, stay in shape, and feel like a part of the community in a relaxed, clean, upscale atmosphere for an affordable price. From tennis, to cardio, to yoga and massages, and of course my weekly Method and Zumba classes, I have found everything I need here — and more, including their babysitting services. Intensity is the best I've experienced in all my 25 years of fitness.

Keep your health on track by joining a one-stop shop fitness club like this. You'll be glad you did, especially during the cold winters when it's hard to stay motivated or exercise outside. Look at it as your new health insurance plan!

Kaia Yoga Complete Wellness Center

kaiayoga.com
Westport, 1200 Post Road
Greenwich, 328 Pemberwick Road at the Mill

Kaia Yoga is another one of my favorite local stops for weekly rejuvenation and fitness. As a busy mom, I love coming here for an hour and taking a Gentle Yoga or Vinyasa Class to re-energize. The family program is like no other, too. My daughter and I have been doing yoga classes here since she was three months old. She loves them! And we always stop by the café afterwards for a smoothie or green juice. My daughter's favorite is the Orange Essence Smoothie made with mangoes, strawberries, bananas and fresh squeezed orange juice.

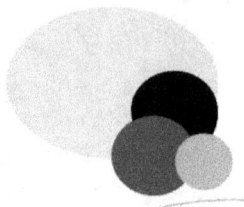

"I am indeed living the lifestyle and not even thinking about it. It has become so natural that when I occasionally slip back to my old ways of eating I am so quickly back on my feet. There is nothing in my fridge or pantry that I am not excited about eating. I take walks in our neighborhood during my lunch and my weekends are filled with hikes and yoga".

~ *Tanya G., Client, Mom, Fashion Designer, Los Angeles, CA*

SLIM AND SEXY TIP #6

Detox Daily With Vibrant Superfoods

Detoxify your body without having to go on a dramatic cleanse or all juice fast by simply adding more rich, satisfying, superfoods into your diet. This is THE secret to significantly fueling your energy, preventing disease, boosting your immune system and turning back the clock.

Action Step:
Make This Work In Your Life NOW!

To detoxify your body the quickest way possible, make it a priority to have a green juice a couple times a week, preferably in the morning or on an empty stomach for maximum absorption. This will take off years! Organic, fresh, non-pasteurized green vegetable juices are one of the number one superfoods and provide an abundance of alkalinity, vitamins, minerals, nutrients and enzymes that hydrate our cells and make us glow from within. They consist of the juices from green vegetables (spinach, kale, celery, cucumber, parsley) and some fruits, like apple or pineapple, ginger and lemon to take away any bitterness from the greens.

If you don't have a juicer at home, you can find a local organic juice bar in your neighborhood that will make one for you. Simply ask for a "green juice" with apple, ginger, etc.

Disease cannot grow in an alkaline environment. If you decrease acidic foods (animal meats, pasteurized cow's dairy, coffee, alcohol, refined sugar, refined flours) and boost alkaline foods (raw vegetables and fruits), you will be amazed when you look in the mirror. You'll see new levels of energy, glowing skin, weight loss, shinier hair, stronger nails, regularity, stabilized moods and a change in your taste buds towards healthier foods. That's a lot of fabulousness for one green juice!

"Okay to Fabulous" Local Resource:

Catch A Healthy Habit
catchahealthyhabit.com
39 Unquowa Rd., Fairfield - 203.292.8190

Start your day with Glen and Lisa, the owners of Catch a Healthy Habit. They make delicious, energizing organic green juices and thick, creamy smoothies that'll jumpstart your day. Try the "Creamsicle" smoothie. It's my absolute favorite. You'll get a different energy boost than your Starbucks coffee. Plus, this small diet modification can take years off your real age.

This cafe showcases all the wonderful options a plant-based diet has to offer. They use superfoods in creative combinations that really pump up your meals, palette and energy levels. I find I always go back for the chia seed pudding, the nori wraps with fig marmalade, avocado and nut cheese, and their meal-sized salads that have add-ins like "rawmesan" (if you're curious, like I was, you've got to try it!), goji berries, avocado and olives. With all of these hydrating, nutrient-rich combinations and flavors, you won't believe you're eating healthy.

Glen and Lisa sell products for your own pantry, like plant-based protein powders for smoothies, crackers, kale chips, onion rings and amazing desserts, like the rich chocolate pudding that my daughter LOVES. All of their menu items and products will inspire your individual efforts in your own kitchen. Glen, Lisa and their staff believe in educating the community about living a plant-based lifestyle. I highly recommend checking out some of their free events, classes and lectures.

"Spend as

much time

enjoying

the meal as

it took to

prepare it."

~ Michael Pollan,
Food Rules, An Eater's Manual

SECTION THREE

HAVE YOUR CAKE AND EAT IT, TOO!

You can finally put to rest the idea that a cleansing, healthy lifestyle is boring and about deprivation. Imagine what it would feel like to have radiant skin, the body and energy levels you've always dreamed of, and be in better shape now than you were in your 20's. All this while still satisfying your cravings and hearty appetite.

You don't have to eat a fat-free or low-calorie artificial snack to count calories and fat grams in your head, just to stay at your ideal weight. <u>Just because it has no calories doesn't mean it's good for you!</u>

Wholesome food with healthy fats and real ingredients enhance our blood, organs and cells, keep us naturally slim, and give our palettes bursts of flavors and the nutrients necessary for our bodies to function with ease and efficiency.

SLIM AND SEXY TIP #7

Rev Up Late-Night Snacks

Instead of giving in to chips, pizza, ice cream, baked goods or candy that can make you feel bloated, falsely energized and contribute to poor digestion (which leads us down a path of ailments, rather than vibrancy), add in more wholesome foods to your diet when a late night craving creeps up on you. It's okay!

Cravings are the body's way of telling us it needs attention. Don't ignore them. Simply make better choices when cravings come up. Otherwise, they will get you. We all know if we ignore them, they come back with a vengeance and cause us to eat large quantities of things we don't want to eat.

Action Step:
Make This Work In Your Life NOW!

To improve your cravings when they hit, and to keep your fabulous body and positive attitude all year round, make upgraded replacements. Instead of fat-free, sugar-free cookies, a pint of ice cream, or a refined sugar-loaded cookie (the size of your head), grab for these delicious, health-generating and decadent snacks instead. As with anything too good, remember to enjoy in moderation:

Vanilla Bean Coconut Milk Ice Cream from **Purely Decadent, SO Delicious** is a wonderful dairy and soy-free ice cream sweetened with agave, a low glycemic natural sweetener. It's rich and creamy and great for those with dairy sensitivities. Häagen-Dazs lovers, be prepared for a delightful surprise.

Top the ice cream with this easy and delicious **chocolate sauce:** Simply mix 2 tablespoons agave syrup and 1 tablespoon dark cocoa powder until dark and creamy. Dip fresh chopped fruit or Brazil nuts into the chocolate sauce and get cozy with your favorite book or magazine after a healthy dinner.

If ice cream isn't your thing, try a **TLC cookie** or two from **Kashi** (I like the dark chocolate chip). They contain whole grain flour and carob, two nutrient-dense, whole ingredients. Another late-night favorite is **stovetop popcorn.** Add olive oil, sea salt and nutritional yeast while it's still warm (a great source of vitamin B) and you'll have a guilt-free, "cheesy" flavored treat for movie watching.

Make these easy upgrades and you'll feel like a part of life – not like a restrictive "dieter" eating empty calories and feeling left out.

"Okay to Fabulous" Local Resource:

Whole Foods
Darien, 150 Ledge Road - 203.662.0577
Fairfield, 350 Grasmere Avenue - 203.319.9544
Westport, 399 Post Road - 203.227.6858
Greenwich, 90 E Putnam Avenue - 203.661.0631

Mrs. Green's Natural Market
Fairfield, 1916 Post Road - 203.255.4333
Stamford, 960 High Ridge Road - 203.329.1313

You can pick up **SO Delicious** ice cream or the **TLC Kashi** cookies at your local Whole Foods or Mrs. Greens Natural Markets. I also love **Pamela's** shortbread cookies and **Pure** whole grain cookies (thepurestfood.com). While you're in these sections at your health food store, check out the other flavors of **So Delicious** ice cream like, cookie dough, chocolate, and mocha almond fudge.

After a long day, I might have a large green salad and then indulge in a cup of coconut ice cream drizzled with the healthy **chocolate sauce** (p. 29). And on special occasions, like birthdays or holidays, I'll add in a cookie, too. Heaven!

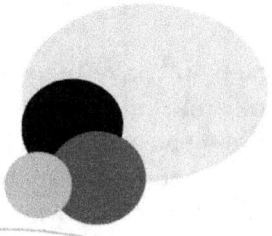

"I want you to know how big an impact you've had on my life in a few short weeks. I'm a changed person – you've taught me so much about foods and the effects on my body. Now, I can have a fruit shake for breakfast, a meatless dinner with veggies and grains, and a salad for lunch. Completely satisfying and I feel so energetic. Also, after swallowing the smallest bite of a sugary birthday cake for an office mate the other day, I not only realized how truly awful it tasted, but also how awful it would make me feel later. Now, that's what I call an education and you are to be thanked, Lisa."

~ Cindy R., Client, Mom, PR Consultant, New York City

SLIM AND SEXY TIP #8

Get Fat and Flavor Crazy

You won't have to sacrifice flavor in order to feel and look amazing. You will still get to enjoy the basic tastes every balanced meal has to offer: sweet, salty, fatty, acidic, sour and spicy by having condiments in your kitchen that instantly provide bursts of flavor without ruining your health.

With a new and improved pantry, you will soon be picking from a range of flavors that support good health. You don't have to give up fat or flavor or your unique, sassy style to look and feel fabulous when you're reaching for natural, fresh flavors fit for human consumption. Forget artificial dyes, corn syrup, sweeteners, flavor crystals, and all the other mystery ingredients we see on food labels in the major grocery stores. Natural condiments are the way to eat healthy and still enjoy the flavors that you love.

Action Step:
Make This Work In Your Life NOW!

You're not a boring person, so why would you eat boring food? And let's face it ladies, the flavors we crave the most are sugar, fat, and salt, am I right? Here are some basic ingredients to use in recipes that will satisfy your cravings whether you are at home, work or on-the-go. Look for snacks with these ingredients in them and use them in your everyday meals while roasting, sautéing, grilling, marinating or blending.

Sweet:
Maple Syrup, Stevia, Raw Honey, Dates, Agave,
Dried Fruits

Salty:
Soy Sauce, Sea Salt, Sea Vegetables (Nori, Dulse)

Fatty:
Raw Nuts, Seeds, Avocado, Cold-Pressed Oils, Coconut
Butter, Organic Butter, Ghee (clarified butter), Olives

Acidic/Sour:
Vinegars, A squeeze of fresh lemon or lime,
fresh citrus juices

Spicy:
Fresh herbs, Curries, Fresh Ginger, Garlic, Cinnamon,
Turmeric, Cayenne

Go to my blog: livewellbydesign.net/blog and
see how these flavors can be used in simple recipes for
ultimate satisfaction, flavor and taste.

"Okay to Fabulous" Local Resource:

The Organic Market
285 Post Rd East, Westport - 203.227.9007

This hidden treasure in Westport will be your "home away from home" if you don't have time to make something for yourself or your family. Or, if you just want to taste some of the best organic, home-made meals, fresh juices and lunches around. Maggie, owner and self-taught food expert, cooks everything from scratch so you don't have to. Forget going to the major grocery store chains that are filled with products with artificial and refined ingredients.

This market has organic soups that include brown rice and vegetable medleys or sweet potato and carrot purees, to gluten-free banana, blueberry muffins made with whole grain flours. Her fresh avocado and homemade mozzarella cheese sandwiches, supersized salads, and hot organic entrees (with fish, beef and veggie options, like stuffed acorn squash) will keep you running back.

I LOVE their ratatouille! I eat it as a side to my piece of salmon and fresh green salad I make at home. I warm up the ratatouille and put grated raw goat's cheese on top right as it comes out of the oven. (**Shiloh Farms Raw Goat's Milk Cheddar Style Cheese** is a good brand available at Organic Market and other health food stores.) This side tastes better and is better for you than any late night pizza.

"Get out of the

supermarket

whenever you can.

You won't find any

high-fructose corn syrup

at the Farmer's Market or

elaborately processed

food lists with long lists of

unpronounceable ingredients."

~ **Michael Pollan,**
Food Rules, An Eater's Manual

SLIM AND SEXY TIP #9

Think Smoothies

Smoothies that taste like milkshakes, a frequent part of my diet? What? Drink smoothies and you'll be giving your body a burst of antioxidants, fiber and live nutrients to give you energy when you need it most, like during a long morning of errands, an outdoor playdate or before a big presentation at work.

And I don't mean the Jamba Juice kind. I'm talking about the kind made with superfoods and real ingredients that include fruits, greens, coconut water, almond milk and even a supplement here or there, like bee pollen, cacao nibs or maca root for increased energy and libido. Hooray! Let the cleansing, sexy lifestyle begin.

Action Step:
Make This Work In Your Life NOW!

Here's a quick smoothie recipe that will rock all of you chocolate lovers out there. I have it for lunch or as an afternoon snack. It'll take you back to your "Fudge-sicle" days, which I grew up on in the 70's, minus the high-fructose corn syrup. I suggest buying some basic ingredients for your kitchen to make one or two smoothies you love and build your list of ingredients as you go.

To get started, stock your kitchen with bananas, berries, almond milk, cocoa powder, cinnamon, liquid stevia, coconut water, and almond butter and you'll be ready to blend at any given moment.

Fudge-sicle Smoothie

1 1/2 frozen bananas

a few drops liquid stevia

2 tbsp carob or dark cocoa powder

dash or two of cinnamon

one scoop **Sun Warrior Vanilla Protein Powder** (16 grams of plant-based protein per scoop. Available at Catch a Healthy Habit or amazon.com)

1-2 cups almond milk

a dash of vanilla extract

a dash of sea salt (it will bring out the chocolate flavor)

Blend all ingredients in a high-speed blender. Adjust anything to fit your tastes and feel like a kid again!

"Okay to Fabulous" Local Resource:

The Stand Juice Company
thestandjuice.com
Norwalk, 31 Wall Street - 203.873.0414
Fairfield, 87 Mill Plain Road - 203.956.5670

If making a smoothie at home isn't always an option, **The Stand** in Norwalk and Fairfield offers a range of delicious, nutrient-dense smoothies. My favorite is the "Hempster" made with apple, banana, cinnamon, hemp protein and almond milk. The hemp seeds are a healthy fat that contain protein and digest slowly in the body for prolonged energy.

Their homemade chocolate almond milk tastes like a dessert. I sip on this as a treat throughout my workdays for extra energy. It definitely doesn't last very long in my fridge!

If you're doing errands and don't have time to sit down for lunch, a smoothie from The Stand is a great option that will keep you satisfied until dinner.

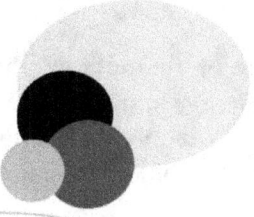

"You helped me sort out a few meal plans and healthy desserts that made the biggest shift for me. And your e-newsletter with new recipes have been a HUGE help! Your protein smoothies are delicious. In the past I would get bored with eating the same old salads and go back to eating unhealthy foods, but you've given me so many choices to make healthy eating fun, easy and really tasty. Those "last five pounds" that I haven't been able to lose for the "last ten years" have literally fallen off me without me even thinking about it."

~ *Tammy H., Mom, Creative Director, Westport, CT*

SLIM AND SEXY TIP #10

Don't Go Without Desserts

One of the most exciting parts about this lifestyle is not having to give up sweets in order to lose weight or reach specific health goals. This news brings joy to many women, including myself!

Indulge in sweets by replacing refined sugars with pure maple syrup, thick raw honey, agave, raw cocoa and dried dates as sweetening agents in recipes. It's a wonderful way to have sweets in nourishing ways. You can have your cake and eat it, too.

Refined sugars and carcinogenic saccharin-laden packets falsely lure you into a sense of "sweet" security while they toxify your cells. By avoiding these sweeteners, your body will thrive and the pounds will drop off. Not to mention your eyes and skin will take on a new glow.

Life is meant to be sweet! Enjoying a naturally sweet treat at the end of a meal is okay in moderation, if you desire. Ladies, making this refinement in your diet is a GAME CHANGER.

Action Step:
Make This Work In Your Life NOW!

Start by stocking organic dark or raw chocolate (70% or more cocoa content) in your kitchen. Dark chocolate is a perfect, on-the-go, low glycemic snack loaded with antioxidants. Add **Larabars** to your kitchen, too. They are a chewy, fruit, nut and spice bar that come in flavors like Coconut Cream Pie, Pecan Pie and Carrot Cake. Another thing to try is high-quality spelt or whole grain cookies sweetened with pure maple syrup (like **Kollar** brand available at **kollarcookies.com**).

You don't have to give in to refined cookies, cake or candy bars just because they're in the cupboards, at business meetings, airports or social events. Finding them or bringing them with you just takes a little practice and planning.

When you're low on energy and the smell of baked goods is calling your name, grab for these types of snacks instead. You won't experience elevated blood sugar levels, which means no energy crash later, and no weight gain from the extra "junk" that gets stored as fat when it's not metabolized properly. That's pretty fabulous.

"Okay to Fabulous" Local Resource:

One Lucky Duck

oneluckyduck.com
Gramercy Park, 125 E 17th St., New York, NY
Chelsea Market, 425 W 15th St,. New York, NY

One of my favorite places both online and at the actual store in New York City is **One Lucky Duck**. When I first went there to shop, my whole perspective on desserts changed. It's amazing what sweet creations can be made with whole, raw sweeteners. I love their chocolate and blonde macaroons made with organic dried coconut, raw agave, coconut oil, vanilla extract, Himalayan salt, cocoa powder, and maple syrup. My tip to you, you may just want to order more than you think you'll need. They are that decadent and good.

Raw Chocolate Love

rawchocolatelovenyc.com

This was my first piece of raw chocolate that I ever experienced. After sampling many kinds of raw dark chocolate over the years, this brand has always remained my #1 favorite.

It's a high quality, dairy-free dark chocolate, made with raw and organic ingredients and superfoods. Honestly, it's too good to be true. That's all I'm going to say. My favorite flavors? Dark Love (plain), Fresh Coconut Love and Peanut Butter Love. Great for travel, as an afternoon snack, or as a perfect ending to a meal with a cup of herbal tea.

Izzie B's Cupcakes

Bakery in Norwalk – 203.810.4378
ibcakes.com for information, orders and select
retail stores

These gluten-free, sugar-free cupcakes are a hit in our home and with guests. I almost don't want to tell anyone what they were made of because you won't believe a treat can taste so yummy without all the refined sugar and preservatives. I just serve them and don't say a word. I let people's taste buds be the judge. It's hard to choose between the Pumpkin with Maple Frosting, Vanilla and Chocolate. These were all a hit at my daughter's first birthday, and probably will be for her 2nd, 3rd, 4th, etc.

"If you don't

have time to

be sick,

make time to

be healthy."

~ **Martha Stewart Living,**
SiriusXM Radio

YOUR "OKAY TO FABULOUS" FOOD CHART

When I first started this lifestyle, I thought, oh no, this might be too limiting. Many experts that I respected in my field told me what foods to stay away from for better health, ideal weight, more energy, etc. It sounded something like this: NO white flour, NO white sugar, NO wheat, NO pasteurized cow's dairy, NO soy... oh my goodness, what could I eat? I panicked.

This was the key for me: I didn't get too extreme. I used transitional foods to get healthy gradually. That means I started eating wholesome versions of the refined junk that was keeping me sick and stuck both emotionally and physically. I started eating whole grain pastas and breads instead of white bread and pasta. I switched to natural sweeteners like dried fruits, maple syrup and agave. I made sure I always included fat in my diet from real foods like avocados and olive oil, not from trans fats or saturated fats.

A food chart is what helped me make sense of what foods to eat. I've created one for you to help you see and understand all of the real, whole foods readily available to you for an abundance of flavors, textures and delicious combinations. It will help you create simple meals for home, on-the-go, or when eating out.

Eat these types of foods and use my tips and resources from this book to promote wellness and balance in your body. Say goodbye to premature aging and cellular degeneration that go hand-in-hand with eating packaged, artificial, non-health generating foods.

In this lifestyle, we build meals that are vegetable and fruit-centric no matter where we are. That means about 50% of our meals include fruits and/or vegetables. You can then add other foods and ingredients from the other categories and season them to your liking for added volume, taste, and flavor. Have fun indulging!

For quick, mouth-watering recipes using these food categories, go to: **livewellbydesign.net/blog**

YOUR "OKAY TO FABULOUS FOOD" CHART

ALL FRUITS AND VEGETABLES
Includes all fruits, and starchy vegetables, like
sweet potatoes, peas and butternut squash, AND
non-starchy vegetables, like cucumbers, carrots, broccoli,
dark leafy greens, Brussels sprouts, cauliflower, etc.

PROTEIN
Includes organic chicken, fish, beef,
shellfish, eggs, raw goat cheeses,
organic dairy, etc.

STARCHES
Includes whole grain breads, and pastas,
whole grains (brown rice, millet, quinoa),
sweet potatoes, legumes, cooked corn,
winter squashes, etc.

NUTS, SEEDS, DRIED FRUITS
Includes almonds, walnuts, pecans, raisins,
dates, cranberries, pine nuts, sesame
seeds, pumpkin seeds, etc.

HEALTHY FATS
Includes cold-pressed oils,
avocados, raw nuts and seeds,
organic butter, ghee, nut butters, etc.

YOUR SLIM AND SEXY SHOPPING LIST

Here are a variety of great-tasting items that create fulfilling eating experiences and a lean, healthy body. Add items like this to your pantry and you will be well on your way to getting and staying slim and sexy.

And notice that none of these items say things like fat-free, low-fat or "only 100 calories" on them. Get used to indulging with this new mindset for higher levels of long-term health at your desired weight. Keep this in your purse for a quick reference anytime you're at the store.

YOUR SLIM AND SEXY SHOPPING LIST

- ❑ Fresh Vegetables/Fruits (Go crazy! Experiment. Try new things each week, and remember organic, seasonal & local is best)
- ❑ Raw Goat's or Sheep's Milk Cheeses (Shiloh Farms Brand is good or the cheese departments at your local health store chain, like Whole Foods or Fairway)
- ❑ Fish, Eggs, Chicken or Beef (wild, organic, hormone and antibiotic-free)
- ❑ Almond, Hemp or Rice Milk (original, vanilla or chocolate)
- ❑ Spelt, Kamut and Quinoa Pasta Products
- ❑ Whole Grain Tortillas and Breads
- ❑ Lara Bars
- ❑ Whole Grain Cookies
- ❑ Mary's Gone Crackers
- ❑ Kale Chips
- ❑ Dried Fruits
- ❑ Dijon Mustard
- ❑ Sea Salt
- ❑ Balsamic Vinegar
- ❑ NuNaturals Stevia
- ❑ Agave
- ❑ Organic Butter
- ❑ Olive Oil
- ❑ Tahini
- ❑ Dark Cocoa Powder
- ❑ Tomato Sauce (no sugar)
- ❑ Tamari or Soy Sauce
- ❑ Lemons, Limes
- ❑ Herbs and Spices (i.e.: cinnamon, oregano, basil, mint, nutmeg, ginger)
- ❑ Plenty of Avocados and Bananas
- ❑ Wine, Water, Herbal Teas, Coconut Water
- ❑ Coconut Milk or Goats Milk Ice Creams
- ❑ Raw or Dark Chocolate (70% or more cocoa content)

WORK WITH LISA PRIVATELY

Ready to live a happy, sexy life in a body you love? Then this is the first step:

Schedule a Nutrition Breakthrough Session with me today.

- Discover how your everyday food and lifestyle choices affect your health, family, work and your ability to feel slim, sexy and strong.
- Uncover which nutrition patterns fuel your life goals, which ones sabotage them — and find out what to do about it.
- Outline a custom designed action plan to take charge of your weight, energy, and health issues (without turning your life upside down or giving up your favorite comfort foods).

Just visit my website to sign up today:
livewellbydesign.net/breakthrough.html

If you're finally ready to get slim and sexy and stay that way, I'm ready to show you how.

I can't wait to chat!

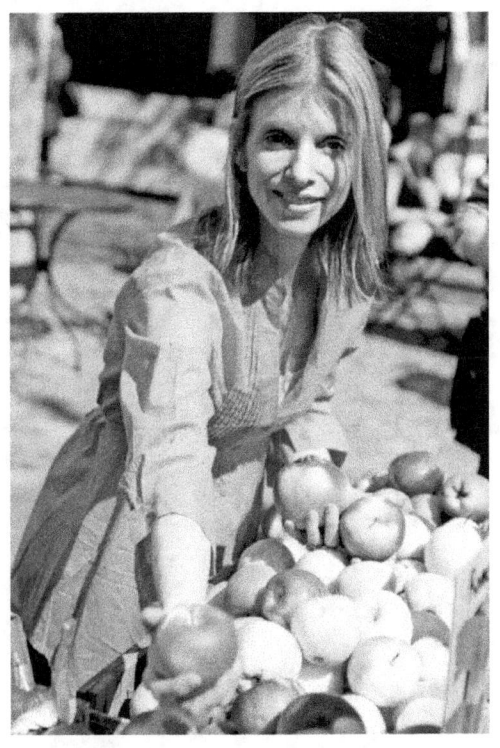

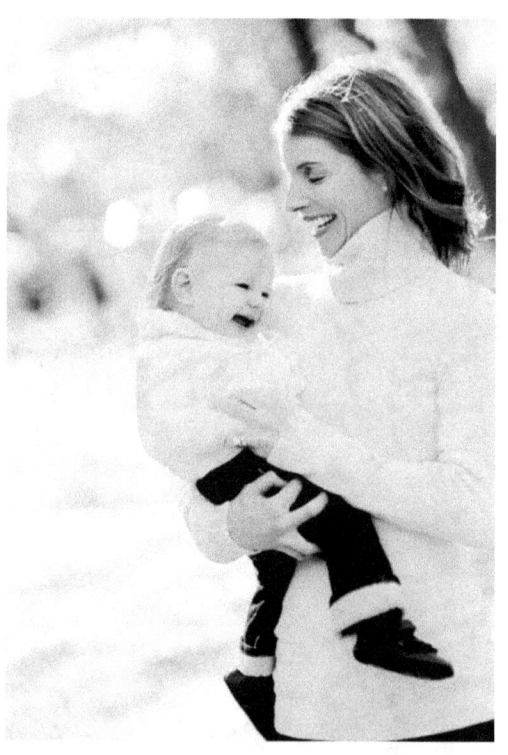

JOIN THE "LIVE WELL BY DESIGN" MOM'S CLUB

If you're ready to live a happy, sexy life in a body you love, turn back the clock, and be your best self to be the best mom, then you'll want to join us.

Where else can you find authentic connections, community and support on the things that really matter to you? I couldn't find it, so I created it!

Join the only mom's club that nourishes your desires for "me time" AND totally inspires you to keep you and your loved ones healthy.

For complete details visit:
livewellbydesign.net/club.html

NOTES:

NOTES:

NOTES:

NOTES:

NOTES: